COPD:
The Eat to Breathe Plan to Feeling Better

COPD:
The Eat to Breathe Plan to Feeling Better

Teri L. Pizza

Copyright © 2017 Teri L. Pizza
All rights reserved.

ISBN: 154116816X
ISBN 13: 9781541168169

Other books by this author:

Simplicity of Fresh Produce
ENJOY! Recipes for Fresh Produce
Joy of Growing Old with God

To God and all my caregivers.

Contents

Forward/Prologue.. xi

Introduction to The Eat to Breathe Plan 1
Eat to Breathe Plan... 5
What You Need for Breakfast................................ 13
What You Need for Your Mid- Morning Snack 15
What You Need at Your Main Meal (Lunch) 17
What You Need for An Afternoon Snack 19
What You Need at Dinner 21
Beverage Recipes 23
Greens Recipes 35
Fruit Recipes 47
Nut & Seed Recipes 59
Protein Recipes.. 71
Vegetable Recipes 91
Whole Grain Recipes 103

Planning to Use The Plan................................... 115
Your Toolbox 117
Sources 121
Support Organizations and Resources Not Listed Elsewhere .. 125
Recipe Index 127
Acknowledgements... 129
About the Author 131

Forward/Prologue

COPD ranks as the third highest cause of death in the United States, killing every four minutes. COPD has killed more American women than breast cancer or diabetes combined (National Center for Health).

The first thing to do if you or a caregiver suspect you have COPD is get tested. Your General Practitioner can order the tests which are simple and noninvasive to determine your diagnosis. Next, if the diagnosis is COPD, get referred to a lung doctor — a pulmonologist. This disease is not medically the same for everyone and should not be treated the same. A specialist will customize a specific treatment for you. Remember, "the sooner, the better," are words to take seriously.

COPD stands for *Chronic Obstructive Pulmonary Disease*. It can include emphysema, chronic bronchitis, refractory asthma and bronchiectasis disorders--disorders that create breathing problems for individuals and make breathing difficult.

COPD is a slow, progressive disease. Progress is marked by four recognized stages with 4 being the most severe. Most sufferers don't get medical help until they are well into double digits age wise. I was 62 when first diagnosed with COPD. Being stubborn, I decided to "make do." When

I was 65 years old, I could barely blow out a candle held in front of my mouth. That's when I got serious and visited a pulmonologist. My FEV1 test came back at 30% (stage 4)!

This book is the result of changes I've made to live better with this disease. I now exercise 4 times a week and use oxygen ***only*** at night. I maintain a prolific writing career as both an author, columnist and sometimes speaker. I remain involved with my church, community and friends. I continue to travel to visit family.

HOWEVER, I almost waited too long to find my way to this "living better, eating better, and feeling better" life. Maybe I wouldn't be on oxygen at all if I had gotten the proper medication and advice sooner. Please don't wait as long as I did. Get checked and begin to live better.

The next thing you can do for yourself is learn what and when to eat! That is what this book is all about. The "Eat to Breathe Plan" in this book can provide a better lifestyle to COPD sufferers. This book will help patients, at any stage, live with their illness in the best possible way.

There's no known cure for COPD but there are things you can do to live and breathe better. The Eat to Breathe Plan is one tool in our toolbox to help us and those we love live better with COPD.

Let food be thy medicine and medicine be thy food. -Hippocrates

Introduction to The Eat to Breathe Plan

Failure to plan is one reason why many people tend to not eat better. We've become a fast-food culture. Instant gratification has invaded our homes as in, "A candy bar will satisfy my hunger." So, the first and best thing we can do is PLAN how and what we are going to eat at any given time of the day or even for a whole week!

Portion size is another important factor to pay attention to as respiratory-impaired patients. When we eat, our stomachs expand to accommodate the food. The stomach presses on the diaphragm. The diaphragm pushes upward, pressing on the lungs and diminishing lung capacity. Keeping portions small is a key component to breathing easier.

What is the proper amount the average person should eat? The newest suggestion is two cups of food, three times a day. [Harvard T.H. Chan School of Public Health; Healthy Eating.org and Healthy Living Plate."] Half of this *plate* (1 cup of food) should consist of fruit and vegetables. The other half (another cup of food) is evenly divided between whole grains and a protein food item.

That is what is recommended for normal, healthy people *without* pulmonary restrictions. COPD patients should eat smaller meals and supplement with snacks. The chapters in this book tell you exactly what types of food are needed each day, broken down into each meal and snack time **plus** provide recipes and suggestions to get you started on the right track.

As pulmonary patients, it's important to eat iron and protein each day. Our goal is 40-52 grams protein and eight milligrams of iron per day.

Protein gives us energy and, along with iron, produces antibodies that fight infection. Dr. Oz put it this way, "Protein is vital to your health.... Consider it the fuel you need to keep all parts of your engine running optimally."

Iron is critical. Too little iron can cause anemia (often found in the elderly) and increase risk of illness. The University of Wisconsin Health Department suggests people age 50 and older get 8 milligrams a day. Warning: "Large amounts of iron can be toxic." Ask your doctor to recommend an iron intake appropriate for you.

Notice we haven't talked about calories. If you are overweight, losing some pounds will help you breathe easier. The options and recipes in this book will help you to do that almost without trying.

The amazing truth is that COPD patients tend to burn ten calories per breath per day! In fact, weight loss is a concern for 40-70 percent of COPD patients. Pounds will just fall off with light exercise and by following the meal plan outlined in this book. If it changes too quickly, a visit to your doctor is in order.

Michael Greger, doctor and author of New York Times best seller, *How Not to Die*, has produced a "Daily Dozen". You can Google his chart at NutritionFacts.org. His dozen includes eleven food groups a healthy person should consume each day. To complete his dozen, he added exercise as his twelfth component, always encouraged especially for COPD patients. (Strong chest muscles help our lungs work better.)

I've modified Dr. Greger's "dozen" for COPD/respiratory patients. This Eat to Breathe Plan gives the COPD patient:

- The recommended servings for each food category.
- Explanations why certain foods are important to lung health.
- Cautions on what food may cause breathing problems.
- Suggestions and recipes for each meal or snack.

This plan will help you or someone you love, breath and live better!

Eat to Breathe Plan

Your Daily Plan

Each day, we need the following food groups in our bodies to help us breathe and function better. I am presenting an overview of the plan below. Don't get overwhelmed—it's easier than it looks, just give it a quick scan for now.

Protein: 3 Servings

Lean protein sources are: eggs, beans, legumes, poultry, and grass-fed red meat. Twice a week try to include fresh, cold-water fish, wild-caught salmon, sockeye salmon, anchovies, sardines, mackerel or herring.

> *Avoid cured meat with nitrates. According to Dr. Michael Gregor, it is now believed that, "nitrates in cured meat may mimic the lung-damaging properties of the nitrite by-products of cigarette smoke." (Good news, some companies now offer nitrate-free cold cuts, sold in most groceries.)*
>
> *Shrimp, because of sulfites, narrow bronchial passages. Fried foods that result in acid reflux response should be avoided.*
>
> *If using canned beans, rinse them to reduce sodium levels. If you find you're not able to get enough protein, add protein powder to soups,*

sauces or smoothies. Daily protein grams should be between 40 & 52 for those over fifty years of age. Strive for 15 grams of protein per meal and 3-5 per each snack.

Fruit: 4 Servings A Day

Fresh or frozen fruits. Try to make one a serving of berries. Note: "There is a difference between eating (which lessens the risk of diabetes) and drinking a berry."

Avoid large amounts of citrus which can trigger acid reflux. Hint, shop the produce department or salad bar for packaged and pre-prepped produce.

Greens: 2 Servings A Day

Mixed green salads are a good choice. Think outside the box and add some turnip greens, dandelion, beet greens, etc., to your next salad.

Avoid kale, Bok Choy, and cabbage, all of which are in the cruciferous family—see below.

Vegetables: 3 Servings A Day

Vegetables with the most protein include spinach, peas, corn, and potatoes. (Purple potatoes are now being touted as a super food.)

Avoid cruciferous vegetables such as broccoli, cauliflower, and Brussels sprouts. Cruciferous vegetables, while healthy, can cause gas and expand the stomach. When these vegetables are cooked, the problem is lessened but use them sparingly. Carotene has caused problems for some patients. It's not that you can't eat carrots or sweet potatoes but don't over indulge. Remember, check with your doctor if you experience or are concerned about any of these issues.

Nuts & Seeds: 1 To 2 Tablespoons Sprinkled On Or Added To Your Food Twice A Day

Flaxseed and nut butters also fall into this category. There seems to be no item in this category that is taboo, unless you have an allergy.

> *Avoid overly salted items. Salty food retains water, making it hard to breath. We only need 1 ½ teaspoons of salt to meet our daily recommended value! Use caution if you use salt substitutes, their ingredients may interact with medications. Check with your doctor.*

Whole Grains: 3 Servings A Day

Good grains include oat, bulgur, millet, quinoa, even orzo and Arborio. Breads should be made from whole grains. Brown rice is better than white. Pasta made with whole wheat is another way to get the needed grains.

Herbs & Spices: Some At Each Meal

Try for a teaspoon at each meal. (Instead of buying fresh herbs, buy the plant for close to the same price. Place on a window sill, water when it starts to wilt and enjoy throughout the year.)

Why all these green things? Well, they can make you better! It's true. A 2010 study showed that COPD's progression was halted when subjects consumed fruit and vegetables over a 3-year period of time. Not only did it not get worse, it even improved a little! *(European Respiratory Journal, 2010.)*

Beverages/Liquids: 6 ½ Servings A Day

Water and other liquids for hydration are crucial. Liquids loosen phlegm, thin mucus and keep airways supple. Some health care providers recommend starting each day with an 8-ounce glass of water. Add 5 more (8-ounce servings), one after each meal and snack. The Cleveland Clinic recommends drinking your beverage after meals instead of before or during so that you do not feel too full.

The best beverages for COPD patients are non-caffeinated liquids. A 4-ounce glass of juice is also recommended. Luckily your intake of fluid can be augmented with soups and most fruits. Caution: If you retain water, follow your doctor's recommendations.

Nutritional experts have selected these juices as the five best: purple grape juice, cranberry juice, pomegranate juice, grapefruit juice, and orange juice. (Dr. Greger considers the "best fruit juice is the one inside a whole fruit." Something to keep in mind.)

Avoid carbonated beverages that can activate acid reflux and vegetable juice drinks that contain salt and a lot of beta-carotene. Reduce the use of caffeine. Substitute red wine for white wine that contains sulfites. Try to eliminate beer because of bloating.

NOTE: The plan is purposely low in fat, salt, sugar, and white flour. The plan is high in the best nutrients to help you breathe better. One tablespoon of oil per day is best. Recommended oils include olive, coconut oil, butter and sesame seed for high temperature cooking.

Use of dairy products should be limited due to their fat content. Dairy tends to thicken mucus, causing plaque which is problematic for lungs. Use low-fat, sweet acidophilus or lactose-reduced milk, low-fat yogurt and hard cheeses instead.

Don't get panicky after reading the "avoid" paragraphs. There's plenty of food left to put color in your cheeks as well as a smile on your face!

The point of this plan is to reduce complications and ease symptoms so you have a more vital existence. "When it comes to COPD, every calorie should contribute to your well-being." (Cindy Reyes, "Foods that Worsen COPD", *Everyday Health Magazine*.)

COPD sufferers need to eat less, per meal, because of what I term the "full tummy phenomenon" or FTP. Starting today, begin to listen to your body, let it tell you what your "less" feels like. For me, when I over eat, I get bloated, my chest heaves slightly and I tend to gasp more often for a deep breath. The Eat to Breathe Plan takes the three squares-a-day thinking and renames it: 3 meals + 2 snacks per day. Again, so our stomachs don't expand (aka FTP).

The plan includes a number of servings from each of the major food groups: Protein, Fruit, Greens, Vegetables, and Whole Grains.

What is your serving size? The perception of the traditional 3 meals a day needs to change. Breakfast, lunch and dinner (with dinner being the largest) will no longer work.

Now, breakfast and lunch need to become the largest meals. Smaller portions, at each meal, sprinkled every few hours with a snack, is ideal. This change allows us time when we are most active to "work off the food" so our breathing capacity isn't compromised.

We need to meet our protein and iron requirements. *When using recipes, some will include ingredients that fulfill other food types recommended for that meal.*

I suggest you begin with a total food volume of 1 ½ cups each for breakfast, lunch and dinner. Don't fret, you get to eat another meal/snack in about two hours. At snack time, try for a total food volume equal to ½ cup to ¾ cup. (See how we're getting our 2+ cups of food per the "Healthy Living Plate" I wrote about in the introduction?) If you feel full or have breathing issues, reduce your food volume by ¼ cup per meal. *Never eliminate a category, just eat less of it for that meal.*

As you taste "good for you" food you'll soon realize that eating to breathe doesn't mean boring food. Once you begin to try the recipes included, you'll agree they are the opposite of boring.

To help you, palate-pleasing recipes, which focus on a particular element of your diet, are included after the meal recommendations. For instance: Stuck for a protein ingredient? Flip to the PROTEIN RECIPES chapter and select from any listed. Do the same if you need an idea or recipe for any of the other categories.

There's a recipe chapter for each essential food to make it easier to follow your plan and feel better. Just remember these three things: what, how much and, when to eat it. It's all listed on the following page:

THE DAILY
EAT TO BREATHE MENU PLAN

BREAKFAST: Protein, Fruit, Whole Grain, Juice and Coffee, Tea or Water

MID-MORNING SNACK: Fruit, Whole Grain, Nuts & Seeds, Vegetable and Water

LUNCH (MAIN MEAL): Protein, Fruit, Greens, Whole Grain and Water

AFTERNOON SNACK: Vegetable, Fruit, Greens, Nuts & Seeds and Water

DINNER: Protein, Vegetable and Beverage (Wine) and Water

**Liberal use of herbs and spices
(other than salt) are encouraged at each meal.**

What You Need for Breakfast

PROTEIN	FRUIT	WHOLE GRAINS	BEVERAGE
1st of 3 DAILY SERVINGS	1st of 4 DAILY SERVINGS	1st of 3 DAILY SERVINGS	Water, tea, or coffee and juice.

To help you, I've relisted the information from Your Daily Plan below:

Protein—begin with a heaping 1/3 cup serving and adjust as needed.

Lean protein sources are: eggs, beans, legumes, poultry, and grass-fed red meat. Twice a week try to include fresh, cold-water fish, wild-caught salmon, sockeye salmon, anchovies, sardines, mackerel or herring. Flip to the *Protein Recipes* chapter to find some that work for you.

Fruit—begin with a heaping 1/3 cup serving and adjust as needed.

Fresh or frozen fruits. Try to have one serving of berries each day. Note: Bored with that handful of fruit or bowl of berries? Flip to the *Fruit Recipes* chapter to find some that work for you.

Whole Grains—begin with a heaping 1/3 cup serving and adjust as needed.

Good grains include oat, bulgur, millet, quinoa, even orzo and Arborio. (Make a little extra and set aside. Use it later at lunch to fulfill this requirement.) Flip to the chapter, *Whole Grain Recipes* to find one that works for you.

Breads should be whole grain. Brown rice is better than white and whole-wheat pasta is another way to get the grains you need.

What You Need for Your Mid-Morning Snack

FRUIT	WHOLE GRAIN	NUTS & SEEDS	VEGETABLE
2nd of 4 DAILY SERVINGS	2nd of 3 DAILY SERVINGS	(1-2 TABLESPOONS) 1st of 2 DAILY SERVINGS	1st of 3 DAILY SERVINGS

Plan to eat about 3/4 cup of food, along with 8 ounces of water. An easy suggestion might be leftovers from a prior meal. To help you, I've relisted the information from Your Daily Plan below:

Fruit—begin with a ¼ cup serving and adjust as needed.
Fresh or frozen fruits; try to make one a serving of berries.

Whole Grains—begin with a ¼ cup serving and adjust as needed.
Good grains include oat, bulgur, millet, quinoa, even orzo and Arborio. Whole grained bread toast is a good option.

Nuts & Seeds—serving size is (1 to 2 tablespoons) can be sprinkled or added to food.

Flaxseed and nut butters also fall into this category. There seems to be no item in this category that's taboo. Ideas can be found in the *Nuts & Seed Recipes* chapter.

Vegetables – begin with an ¼ cup serving and adjust as needed.

Vegetables with the most protein include spinach, peas, corn, and potatoes (purple potatoes are now being touted as a super food). Grocers now precut veggies (and fruit) to make them even easier to plate. Or, shop the salad bar.

[One modification from The Daily Dozen was to add an extra serving of "other vegetables" as a substitute for the one serving of raw cruciferous vegetables he recommends. Again, the recipe chapters can help you find something if you're stumped on what to fix.]

What You Need at Your Main Meal (Lunch)

PROTEIN	FRUIT	GREENS	WHOLE GRAINS
2nd of 3	3rd of 4	1st of 2	3rd of 3
DAILY SERVINGS	DAILY SERVINGS	DAILY SERVINGS	DAILY SERVINGS

Plan for four heaping 1/3 cups servings from the above food groups.

Flip the script. Begin to entertain at lunchtime. Check out the recipe chapters for options. Serve flavored water, coffee, tea, or a light red wine for a beverage. If entertaining, wait to serve fruit. (Your company will have dessert but we'll be having our afternoon fruit snack!)

To help you, I've relisted the information from Your Daily Plan below:

Protein—begin with heaping 1/3 cup serving and adjust if necessary.

Lean protein sources are: eggs, beans, legumes, poultry, and grass-fed red meat. Twice a week try to include fresh, cold-water fish, wild-caught salmon, sockeye salmon, anchovies, sardines, mackerel or herring.

Fruit—begin with a heaping 1/3 cup serving and adjust as needed.

Fresh or frozen fruit; try to make one a serving of berries. Note: "There is a difference between eating (which lessens the risk of diabetes) and drinking a berry.

Greens—begin with a heaping 1/3 cup serving and adjust as needed.

Mixed green salads are a good choice. Think outside of the box and add some turnip greens, dandelion, beet greens, etc.

Whole Grains—begin with a heaping 1/3 cup serving and adjust as needed.

Grains include oat, bulgur, millet, quinoa, even orzo and Arborio. Breads should be made of whole grain. Brown rice is better than white and pasta made with whole wheat is another way to get the grains needed.

What You Need for An Afternoon Snack

VEGETABLE	FRUIT	GREENS	NUT & SEEDS
2nd of 3	4th of 4	2nd of 2	2nd of 2
DAILY SERVINGS	DAILY SERVINGS	DAILY SERVINGS	DAILY SERVINGS

A simple snack could be asparagus spears with grapefruit sections and baby spinach leaves on a platter served with a sesame seed vinaigrette. Or, a diced avocado with shredded lettuce and poppy seed dressing. Make it even more memorable by using one of the recipes suggested for each type of food.

One cup to ¾ cup total food along with an 8-ounce glass of water should be all you need.

To help you, I've relisted the information from Your Daily Plan below:

Vegetables—begin with a ¼ cup serving and adjust as needed.

Vegetables with the most protein include spinach, peas, corn, and potatoes (purple potatoes are now being touted as a super food). Grocers now precut them to make them even easier to plate. Or shop the salad bar

Fruit—begin with a ¼ cup serving and adjust as needed.

Fresh or frozen fruit; try to make one a serving of berries.

Greens—begin with a ¼ cup serving and adjust as needed.

Mixed green salads are a good choice. Think outside the box and add some turnip greens, dandelion, beet greens, etc.

Nut & Seeds—serving size is 1 to 2 tablespoons sprinkled on top or added to food.

There seems to be no item in this category that's taboo.

What You Need at Dinner

PROTEIN	VEGETABLE	BEVERAGE:
3rd of 3	3rd of 3	Water
DAILY	DAILY	and Wine, if
SERVINGS	SERVINGS	desired

Because of our disability, dinner can no longer be a large plate of food. We've eaten well throughout the day when we've been at our busiest and most active. Now comes evening when we are more sedate. We need to decrease our food volume. The recommendation is 1 cup of food.

We might want to eat a smaller amount of something from earlier in the day. Soups and salads (something we might have thought of as a lunch item in the past) are a good idea for this time of day.

With that in mind, some vegetable soup or a salad with added protein and a beverage might be all that's needed. To help you, I've relisted the information from Your Daily Plan below:

Protein — begin with a ½ cup serving and adjust as needed

Lean protein sources are: eggs, beans, legumes, poultry, and grass-fed red meat. Twice a week try to include fresh, cold-water fish, wild-caught salmon, sockeye salmon, anchovies, sardines, mackerel or herring.

Vegetables—begin with a ½ cup serving and adjust as needed.

Try to eat the vegetables with the most protein: spinach, peas, corn, and potatoes.

Beverages/Liquids:

Water and other liquids for hydration are crucial to loosen phlegm, thin mucus and keep your airways supple. Yes, you can have a glass of red wine with dinner (but don't overdo it or you may activate acid reflux).

Beverage Recipes

Banana-Berry Smoothie
English Wassail
Fresh Lemonade or Limeade
German Chocolate Café au Lait
Kiwi Banana Shake for 2
Mulled Wine
Piña Colada Slush
Raspberry Smoothie
Rosy Cranberry Punch
Wild Plum Tea

Banana-Berry Smoothie
Adapted from *Cooking Light Cookbook*

Also, fulfills fruit requirement.

¾ c. cranberry juice
⅔ c. plain low-fat yogurt
1 med. ripe banana, peeled & sliced
1 c. crush ice

Combine juice, yogurt and banana in blender; cover and process until smooth. Add ice and process until smooth. Serve immediately.
Makes 3 cups.

Protein 3
Iron 0

English Wassail

Adapted for stove-top cooking; inspired by *White Westinghouse Microwave Oven Cookbook*

Also, fulfills fruit and herb/spice requirement.

1 qt. apple cider
1 Granny Smith apple, cut-up
½ c. brown sugar
½ c. orange juice
2 Tbsp. lemon juice
2 cinnamon sticks
1 tsp. allspice
½ tsp. ground cloves
¼ tsp. nutmeg

Combine all ingredients in 3-quart saucepan.
Heat on medium-high just until boiling or until temperature reaches 150-160-degrees.
Serve immediately.
Makes 8-10 servings.

Protein 1.2g
Iron 0.3mg

Fresh Lemonade Or Limeade
Adapted from *Better Homes and Gardens New Cook Book*

4 c. water
4-5 fresh lemons or limes, juiced to equal 1 cup juice
⅔ c. sugar
Ice cubes

In pitcher, combine water, juice and sugar. Stir until sugar dissolves. Serve immediately or chill for later use.
Makes 5 (8-oz) servings.

Protein 0.3g
Iron 0.3mg

German Chocolate Café Au Lait

From *Light & Luscious*

¼ c. sugar
2 Tbsp. unsweetened cocoa
½ c. skim milk
2 ½ c. brewed chocolate almond-flavored coffee
½ tsp. coconut extract
½ tsp. almond extract

Combine sugar and cocoa in small saucepan; stir well. Gradually add milk, stirring well.
Place sauce pan over medium heat and cook until sugar dissolves, stir frequently. Remove from heat.
Stir in coffee and extracts.
Pour into individual cups. Serve immediately.
Makes 4 (3/4-cup) servings.

Protein 2g
Iron 0.5mg

Kiwi Banana Shake For 2

From *ENJOY! Recipes for Fresh Produce*

Also, fulfills fruit requirement.

1 ½ c. ice
¼ tsp. vanilla
2 kiwi
2 bananas, chunked

Combine all ingredients together in a blender and purée until it is the consistency you enjoy.
Yummy!

Protein 1g
Iron 0.3mg

Mulled Wine

Adapted for stove-top cooking; inspired by *White Westinghouse Microwave Oven Cookbook*

Also, fulfills herb/spice requirement.

1 qt. red wine
2 ½ c. orange juice
¾ c. sugar
½ c. lemon juice
16 whole cloves
2 cinnamon sticks
1 lemon, sliced

Combine all ingredients except lemon in 3-quart sauce pan.
Cook over medium-high heat 12-14 minutes or until steaming but not boiling.
Garnish and serve.
Makes 8 servings.

Protein 0.6g
Iron 0.1mg

Piña Colada Slush
From *Light & Luscious*

Also, fulfills fruit requirement.

1 med. banana, peeled & sliced
1 Tbsp. lemon juice
6 oz. (½ of 12-oz. can) frozen pineapple juice concentrate, thawed & undiluted
¼ c. instant nonfat dry milk powder
¼ c. water
¼ c. light rum
2 Tbsp. coconut liqueur
1 tsp. coconut extract
Crushed ice

Combine banana and lemon juice; toss gently to coat.
Place banana slices on baking sheet. Cover and freeze 1 hour or until firm. Combine banana, pineapple juice concentrate, dry milk, water, rum, coconut liqueur and extract in blender; cover and process until smooth. Add enough ice to make 4 cups; cover and process until slushy.
Pour slush into glasses. Serve immediately.
Makes 4 (1-cup) servings.

Protein 3.5g
Iron 0.1mg

Raspberry Smoothie
From *realsimple.com*

Also, fulfills fruit (berry), herb/spice requirements.

1 lg. banana, sliced
½ c. frozen raspberries
¼ c. almond milk
2 tsp. honey
¼ tsp. vanilla
Pinch ground cinnamon

Blend banana, raspberries, almond milk, honey, vanilla and cinnamon until smooth and frothy.

Makes 2 servings.

Protein 14g
Iron 2.5mg

Rosy Cranberry Punch

Adapted for stove-top cooking; inspired by *White Westinghouse Microwave Oven Cookbook*

Also, fulfills herb/spice requirement.

1 qt. cranberry juice
1 qt. apple juice
2 Tbsp. lemon juice
2 Tbsp. sugar
4 cinnamon sticks, 2" long
¾ tsp. whole cloves
1 lemon, halved and sliced very thin.

Combine all ingredients, except lemon, in 3-quart sauce pan. Cover and cook over medium-high heat for 20 minutes; stir and simmer an additional 10 minutes until flavors are well blended.
Remove spices with slotted spoon.
Garnish by floating lemon slices on top of each serving of punch.
Makes 14 (½ cup) servings.

Protein 1.1g
Iron 0.3mg

Wild Plum Tea

From Chef Kacy Rothwell, Wild Plum Tea Room, Gatlinburg, TN for St. Mary's Catholic Church's, *From Thy Bounty* cookbook

Also, fulfills herb/spice (tea) requirement.

4 family-size tea bags
2 c. sugar
2 c. orange juice
½ c. lemon juice

Boil 1 quart of water. Steep tea bags for 10 minutes.
In small saucepan, combine sugar with 2 cups of water and boil until sugar is completely dissolved.
Once tea bags have steeped, remove them and add the sugar water, orange and lemon juice.
Makes 1 gallon of tea.

Negligible Protein & Iron

Greens Recipes

Arugula with Plum Sauce
Baked Vegetable Omelet
Beet Greens Side Dish
Fruit Salad with Peanut Butter Dressing
Granny's Radicchio Apple & Celery Root Salad
Kale & Quinoa Salad
Quinoa & Honey Beet Salad
Spinach Carrot Salad
Spinach Tacos
Spring Green & Bean Salad

Arugula With Plum Sauce

From *countryliving.com*

Also, fulfills vegetable and herb/seed requirements.

2 c. pitted plums, roughly chopped
½ c. extra-virgin olive oil
4 Tbsp. white balsamic vinegar
1 tsp. fresh tarragon, chopped
1 tsp. scallions, sliced (white only)
1 tsp. fennel seeds, toasted
Salt & pepper, to taste

Mix all together and marinate for 15 minutes. Spoon over arugula or grilled lamb chops.

Protein 1.5g
Iron 0.5mg

Baked Vegetable Omelet

Also, fulfills protein and herb/spice requirements.

Extra-virgin olive oil for brushing
8 lg. eggs
⅛ c. all-purpose flour
1 ½ Tbsp. + ½ tsp. fresh thyme leaves, chopped
1 tsp. coarse salt
¼ red onion, thinly sliced
1 ½ oz. spinach or kale, stemmed to make 1 ½ cups.

Preheat oven to 325-degrees. Place oven rack in upper third of chamber. Brush a 9x13 rimmed baking sheet with oil. Line with parchment; brush parchment with oil.
Whisk eggs in bowl until combined, then slowly whisk in flour, thyme and salt until smooth. Pour onto prepared baking sheet. Sprinkle with red onion and tuck in greens.
Bake until puffed and golden, about 15-20 minutes. Serve warm or at room temperature; cut into squares.
Makes 6 servings.

Protein 12g
Iron 1.8mg

Beet Greens Side Dish
From *ENJOY! Recipes for Fresh Produce*

Cut leaves from root ball and stalks.
Rinse stalks and leaves 2-3 times.
Steam or boil stems until tender 3-4 minutes.
Add leaves and cook 2-3 minutes more and then drain completely.
Season with salt and pepper, toss with butter or olive oil.
Serve on individual plates with a lemon wedge per person.

Protein 4g
Iron 2.7mg

HINT: ADD BEET GREENS TO YOUR OTHER SALADS AS WELL:
Add the smaller, younger leaves to other lettuce greens and get more nutrition in each meal!

Fruit Salad With Peanut Butter Dressing
From *ENJOY! Recipes for Fresh Produce*

Also, fulfills protein, and fruit requirements.

6 oz. pineapple nectar
¼ c. creamy peanut butter
¾ c. safflower oil
4 c. lettuce
1 c. fresh pineapple chunks
1 c. canned sliced peaches, drained
¾ med. cantaloupe, peeled & wedged

Prepare dressing by mixing pineapple nectar and peanut butter together in blender; process until smooth.
Turn blender to run at high speed and gradually add oil until well blended.
Pour into bowl, cover and chill until ready to serve salad.
Prepare salad by lining dish or individual dishes with lettuce; arrange fruit on top.
To serve, stir dressing and serve on the side with the salad.
Makes 6 servings.

Protein 3g
Iron 1.0mg

Granny's Radicchio, Apple & Celery Root Salad
From *ENJOY! Recipes for Fresh Produce*

Also, fulfills the vegetable and fruit requirements.

½ c. buttermilk
⅓ c. mayonnaise
4 oz. blue cheese, crumbled
¼ tsp. onion powder
½ tsp. salt, divided
⅛ tsp. freshly ground pepper
2 med. heads radicchio, thinly sliced
½ lb. celery root, peeled & thinly sliced
2 Gala apples, thinly sliced
1 Tbsp. fresh lemon juice

In bowl, whisk together buttermilk and mayonnaise; stir in cheese, onion powder, 1/4 teaspoon salt and the pepper. Cover and refrigerate.
Cut sliced celery root and apple into matchsticks.
Toss together radicchio, celery root, apples, lemon juice and remaining salt.
When ready to serve, drizzle half of dressing on top of salad and serve remaining dressing on the side.

Protein 4.7g
Iron 0.2mg

Kale & Quinoa Salad

Adapted from *foodheavenmadeeasy.com*

Also, fulfills whole grain requirement.

3 leaves kale, destemmed
¼ c. quinoa, cooked
½ Tbsp. olive oil

In medium size sauté pan, heat oil. Add kale and cook until wilted. Remove from pan and place in serving bowl.
In same pan, sauté quinoa until fragrant and toasted. Toss in bowl with kale.
Makes 2 servings.

Protein 2.5g
Iron 1.7mg

Quinoa & Honey Beet Salad
From *ENJOY! Recipes for Fresh Produce*

Also, fulfills fruit and whole grain requirements.

2 lbs. baby beets (or 4 medium), peeled & quartered
½ c. balsamic vinegar
1 Tbsp. honey
1 Tbsp. tarragon oil
Salt & pepper, to taste
1 ½ c. quinoa, cooked
2 c. arugula

Place prepared beets on rimmed baking sheet. Combine vinegar, honey, and oil and pour over beets. Season with salt and pepper. Cover and bake at 400° 40-50 minutes or until tender.
Combine cooked quinoa and arugula; place on serving dish. Arrange beets on top of salad and pour roasting juices over all.
Makes 4 servings.

Protein 4g
Iron 1.8mg

Spinach Carrot Salad
From *ENJOY! Recipes for Fresh Produce*

Also, fulfills fruit and vegetable requirements.

1 Tbsp. red wine vinegar
2 tsp. brown sugar
¼ tsp. salt
Pepper, to taste
3 Tbsp. extra-virgin olive oil
1 6-oz. bag pre-washed baby spinach
2 med. carrots, grated
½ c. dried cranberries

Whisk together first three ingredients; whisk in oil. Season with more salt and pepper to taste.
When ready to serve, gently toss in last three ingredients.
Makes 4 servings.

Protein 5g
Iron 0.4mg

Spinach Tacos
Adapted from *foodheavenmadeeasy.com*

Also, fulfills protein and herb/spice requirements.

2 Tbsp. canola oil
6 c. fresh spinach
2 cloves garlic, minced
6 8-inch tortillas
1 c. black beans, rinsed
6 oz. Mixed Mexican cheese, shredded
Pinch paprika, per taco
Pinch sea salt, per taco

Heat oil on medium. Sauté spinach and garlic until spinach is wilted and garlic is softened. Remove from pan, set aside and drain slightly.
In same pan, heat tortillas one at a time.
While tortillas are heating, place black beans in a microwave dish, cover and cook on high 1 minute.
Stuff each tortilla with equal portions of spinach and beans, sprinkle with cheese and top with spices.
Makes 6 tacos.

Protein 9g
Iron 2.9mg

Spring Green & Bean Salad
From *Real Simple* magazine

Also, fulfills protein and herb/spice requirements.

1 5-oz. pkg. mixed spring greens
2 Tbsp. extra-virgin olive oil
1 Tbsp. lemon juice
½ tsp. salt
1 tsp. fresh dill
1 15-oz. can white beans, rinsed & drained
1 sm. shallot, thinly sliced
½ English cucumber, sliced

Toss together the spring greens with the oil, lemon juice, salt and dill. Divide salad among 4 plates and top each with beans, shallot, and cucumber.

Protein 7g
Iron 1.6mg

Fruit Recipes

Apple & Fennel Salad
Cinnamon-Apple Oatmeal
Fruit Salad with Lime
Orzo Salad
Raspberry-Peach Salad
Roasted Apple Sauce
Simple Papaya Avocado Salad
Strawberry Sauce
Zucchini-Apricot/Raisin Salad
Zucchini & Carrot Strands

Apple & Fennel Salad
Inspired by *Cooking Light*

Also, fulfills vegetable and herb/spice requirement.

¾ lb. fennel
1 sm. Red Delicious apple, cored & chopped – do not peel
½ c. seedless red grapes, halved
2 tsp. dried parsley (or 2 Tbsp. fresh parsley, chopped)
3 Tbsp. orange juice
1 Tbsp. extra-virgin olive oil
1 Tbsp. sugar
½ tsp. celery seeds
½ tsp. dry mustard
⅛ tsp. pepper
Butter leaf lettuce

Wash fennel and trim off leaves and rough outer stalks. Cut bulb in half lengthwise, remove core and coarsely chop.
Combine fennel, apple, grapes and parsley.
Combine orange juice and remaining ingredients in saucepan. Cook over medium heat 3 minutes or until thoroughly heated through. Pour over fennel mixture; toss gently. Cover and chill.
Line plates with lettuce; place salad on top.
Makes 4 servings.

Protein 0.9g
Iron 0.6mg

Cinnamon-Apple Oatmeal
Adapted from *Cooking Light Cookbook*

Also, fulfills whole grain requirement.

1 c. water
¾ c. unsweetened apple juice
2 Tbsp. raisins
½ tsp. cinnamon
¾ c. oats, uncooked
2 ½ Tbsp. instant nonfat dry milk powder
1 med. apple, chopped
1 ½ tsp. brown sugar

Combine water, juice, raisins and cinnamon in saucepan; bring to a boil. Add oats and milk powder and cook over medium heat 1 minute for instant oatmeal and 8 minutes for regular oatmeal, stirring occasionally. Cover; let stand 5 minutes.
Add chopped apples; sprinkle with brown sugar.
Makes 4 servings.

Protein 4g
Iron 0.5mg

Fruit Salad With Lime
Adapted from *Cooking Light Cookbook*

Also, fulfills herb/spice requirement.

2 kiwi, peeled & diced
2 oranges, peeled & sectioned
1 c. fresh or thawed frozen strawberries, sliced
2 Tbsp. lime juice
1 Tbsp. + 1 tsp. powdered sugar
¼ tsp. cinnamon

Combine prepared kiwi, oranges and strawberries in medium bowl. Pour lime juice over fruit and toss gently.
Cover and chill at least 3 hours.
Combine sugar and cinnamon; add to fruit mixture and toss well.
Makes 4 servings.

Protein 1.5g
Iron 0.8mg

Orzo Salad

Also, fulfills vegetable and greens requirements.

1 Tbsp. olive oil
½ yellow onion, chopped
1 8-oz. pkg. orzo
2 c. frozen corn
1 c. cherry tomatoes, halved
2 ½ c. baby arugula
1 tsp. salt
½ tsp. pepper
Garnish: lemon zest

Add oil and onion to medium skillet on medium heat and sauté 8 minutes.
Cook orzo according to package directions.
Place corn in microwaveable bowl with 1 tablespoon water, cover and cook 6 minutes, stirring once.
Combine onion, orzo, corn, tomatoes and arugula. Season with salt and pepper. Garnish with lemon zest, if desired and serve.
Makes 4-6 servings.

Protein 8g
Iron 0.7mg

Raspberry-Peach Salad
Adapted from *Cooking Light*

Also, fulfills nut & seed requirement.

1 5-oz. pkg. frozen raspberries, thawed
1 Tbsp. red wine vinegar
4 med. peaches
1 ½ Tbsp. lemon juice
Curly leaf lettuce
¼ c. sliced almonds, toasted

Set aside 12 raspberries, cut in half for garnish.
Place rest of frozen, thawed raspberries in food processor; process until smooth. Add vinegar to puree; stir well, set aside.
Cut peaches in half lengthwise; remove pits. Slice halves lengthwise into ¼-inch thick slices, leaving slices attached ½-inch from stem end. Brush peaches with lemon juice.
Arrange lettuce on 4 individual salad plates. Arrange peaches over lettuce, fanning out slices slightly.
Drizzle each salad with 2 tablespoons raspberry mixture and sprinkle each plate evenly with toasted almonds.
Garnish plates with 3 raspberry halves each, with fresh. Serve immediately. Makes 8 servings.

Protein 2g
Iron 0.5mg

Roasted Apple Sauce
Adapted from *Cooking with Curtis*

4 Honeycrisp apples or any baking apple, cored & quartered into wedges
1 Tbsp. sugar
Water in mister
1 Tbsp. cinnamon

Place oven rack in center of oven and preheat to 400-degrees.
Toss apples with sugar and place apples, cut side down into a 7 x 12-inch baking dish. Mist with water. Bake 55 minutes or until apples are very tender.
When finished baking, cut apples coarsely, sprinkled with cinnamon and serve.
Makes 4 servings.

Protein 1g
Iron 0mg

Simple Papaya Avocado Salad
From *The Baby Cookbook* via Nyteglori

Also, fulfills greens requirement.

1 papaya, cubed
2 avocados, cubed
Mixed greens: spinach and lettuce leaves

DRESSING:
¼ c. lime juice
½ c. olive oil
⅛ tsp. pepper
¼ tsp. salt

Mix dressing ingredients together and gently coat cubed fruit with dressing.
Serve over the greens.
Makes 4 servings.

Protein 5g
Iron 1.2mg

Strawberry Sauce
Adapted from *Cooking Light*

Also, fulfills herb/spice requirement.

2 c. strawberries, sliced
1 c. water
¼ c. sugar
2 Tbsp. cornstarch
¼ tsp. cinnamon
⅛ tsp. ground pumpkin pie spice
Pinch ground cloves
Pinch nutmeg
1 tsp. orange zest
Powdered sugar, optional

Combine strawberries and water in saucepan. Cook over medium heat 6 minutes or until tender. Add sugar, cornstarch, cinnamon, pumpkin pie spice, cloves and nutmeg. Cook, stirring constantly until thickened. Stir in zest.
Serve warm or chilled over pancakes, waffles, French Toast, pound cake or angel food cake; dust with powdered sugar if desired.
[Make Strawberry-Rhubarb sauce by reducing strawberries to 1 cup and adding 1 cup diced rhubarb.]
Makes 2 ¾ cup sauce.

Negligible protein & iron.

Zucchini-Apricot/Raisin Salad
Adapted from *Betty Crocker's New American Cooking*

Also, fulfills the greens, herb/spice and nut & seed requirements.

⅓ c. dried apricots, cut-up (or substitute ⅓ c. raisins)
½ c. water
3 Tbsp. olive oil
2 Tbsp. lemon juice
½ tsp. salt
⅛ tsp. dry mustard
⅛ tsp. paprika
Dash red pepper hot sauce
2 med. zucchini, thinly sliced (about 3 c.)
Lettuce leaves
Roasted, salted pumpkin seeds; optional

Place sliced zucchini in a medium size bowl.
Heat apricots/raisins in water to boiling; remove from heat. Cover and let stand 15 minutes; drain and place in bowl with zucchini.
Whisk together oil, lemon juice, salt, mustard, paprika and hot sauce. Pour over apricots/raisins and zucchini. Toss until evenly coated.
Serve on lettuce leaves; sprinkle with pumpkin seeds, if desired.
Makes 4 servings.

Protein 4g
Iron 3.0mg

Zucchini & Carrot Strands
From *Cooking Light*

Also, fulfills vegetable requirements.

Olive oil cooking spray
1 tsp. olive oil
2 med. carrots, peeled & julienned
¼ c. chicken broth
1 med. unpeeled zucchini, julienned
1 clove garlic, minced
¼ tsp. salt
⅛ tsp. pepper

Coat large nonstick skillet with cooking spray. Add oil; place over medium heat until hot. Add carrot and sauté 1 minute. Add chicken broth and cook 1 minute, stirring occasionally.
Stir in zucchini, garlic, salt and pepper. Cover and cook 3 minutes until vegetables are crisp-tender.
Makes 4 servings.

Protein 1g
Iron 0.6mg

Nut & Seed Recipes

Banana Nut Salad
Couscous Fruit & Vegetable Salad
Farro Salad with Toasted Pecans
Granola
Mary's Roasted Pear Salad
Nutty Orange Pancakes
Raspberry Smoothie Bowl
Roasted Pumpkin Seeds
Roasted Stone-Fruit for 2
Sunflower Poppy Seed Muffins

Banana Nut Salad
From Connie Walker for *ENJOY! Recipes for Fresh Produce*

Fulfills fruit and green requirements.

¾ c. granulated sugar
2 eggs
4 Tbsp. water
2 Tbsp. white vinegar
½ head of iceberg lettuce
6 bananas
¾ c. lightly salted peanuts, chopped

Mix sugar, eggs, water, and vinegar together in sauce pan. Heat on low until boiling. (Remove from heat immediately after boiling.) Cool.
Place a bed of lettuce on each plate. Slice bananas length-wise, peel, and place on top of the lettuce.
Cover bananas with the cooled topping.
Sprinkle with chopped peanuts.
Makes 6 servings.

Protein 7.9g
Iron 1.4mg

Couscous Fruit & Vegetable Salad

Adapted from *The View from Great Island* blog

Also, fulfills herb/spice, fruit, vegetable and whole grain requirements.

1 ½ c. couscous
½ cucumber, peeled & diced
½ med. tomato, diced
¼ c. nuts, chopped: slivered almonds, walnuts, pistachios, pine nut, or pecans
1 7-oz. bag mixed dried fruit, cut-up
¼ c. carrot, peeled & diced (or celery, or bell pepper; diced)
5 black olives, sliced
4 oz. or ½ c. feta cheese
Salt & pepper, to taste

DRESSING:
¼ c. olive oil
Juice of 1 lemon
½ tsp. cinnamon
1 tsp. nutmeg
Pinch salt & pepper, if needed

Prepare couscous according to package directions. Cool under cold water and place in large bowl. Add rest of ingredients; salt and pepper to taste. Mix together dressing ingredients, tasting to tweak as needed. Dress salad, using just enough to flavor, but not drown, ingredients.
Keep, covered for one week in the refrigerator.
Makes 6 generous servings. Can easily be doubled for larger groups.

Protein 6g
Iron 1.1mg

Farro Salad With Toasted Pecans
Adapted from *Southern Living* magazine

Also, fulfills fruit, herb/spice and whole grain requirements.

1 ½ c. farro, uncooked
½ c. pecans, toasted & chopped
½ c. dried cherries
⅓ c. scallions, chopped
¼ c. flat-leaf parsley, chopped
2 Tbsp. lemon juice
2 Tbsp. olive oil
¼ tsp. kosher salt
¼ tsp. pepper
½ cup (4 oz.) Feta cheese, crumbled

Bring a large pot of salted water to a boil over high heat.
Add farro and cook, stirring occasionally, until tender, about 15 minutes. Drain well and rinse under cold water. Shake strainer/colander to remove excess water and transfer to medium bowl.
Add pecans, cherries, scallions, parsley, lemon juice, oil, salt and pepper to the farro. Stir gently until combined.
Fold in feta.
Can be serve chilled or at room temperature.
Makes 6 servings.

Protein 10.6g
Iron 1.4mg

Granola
Adapted from *Betty Crocker's New American Cooking*

Also, fulfills fruit, herb/spice and whole grain requirements.

3 c. oats
2 c. golden raisins
1 c. sunflower nuts
1 c. raw cashews or blanched almonds, coarsely chopped
1 c. coconut flakes
1 c. dried apricots (or apples or pears or mixed fruit), cut-up
½ c. vegetable oil
½ c. honey
1 Tbsp. vanilla
¾ tsp. pumpkin pie spice
½ tsp. salt

Mix oats, raisins, sunflower nuts, cashews, coconut and dried fruit in 4-quart bowl.
Mix together remaining ingredients and pour over oat mixture, tossing until evenly coated.
Spread in 2 ungreased jelly roll pans (Each pan measuring 15 ½" x 10 ½ x1".)
Bake in 325-degree oven, stirring frequently, until golden brown, about 30 minutes. Cool.
Store tightly covered in refrigerator up to 2 months.
Makes 18 half-cup servings.

Protein 11g
Iron 1.9mg

Mary's Roasted Pear Salad
From Mary Miller for *ENJOY! Recipes for Fresh Produce*

Also, fulfills protein (cheese) and greens requirements.

3 red pears, firm
¼ c. pecans or walnuts, chopped
4-oz. Gorgonzola
¼ c. dried cherries
1 head butter lettuce

Prepared Balsamic vinaigrette bottled dressing
Preheat oven to 375°.
Slice pears in half lengthwise; use a melon-baller to remove cores and create a hole for filling. Trim a sliver from bottom side of each pear to help each sit in the baking dish. Bake about 25 minutes until fork tender which depends on ripeness of pears. Set aside and let cool to room temperature. To assemble, tear lettuce into bite size pieces and place on 6 salad plates. Place roasted pear half in center of lettuce. Sprinkle nuts, cherries, and cheese into each pear's hole and let ingredients flow over the pear onto the lettuce. Serve with vinaigrette or drizzle dressing over each salad before serving.
Makes 6 servings.

Protein 6g
Iron 0.6mg

Nutty Orange Pancakes

Adapted from *Better Homes and Gardens New Cook Book*

Also, fulfills juice and protein requirements.

1 c. all-purpose flour
1 Tbsp. sugar
2 tsp. baking powder
½ tsp. baking soda
½ tsp. cinnamon
¼ tsp. salt
1 egg, beaten
1 c. orange juice
2 Tbsp. cooking oil
½ c. walnuts or pecans, finely chopped

In mixing bowl, stir together flour, sugar, baking powder, baking soda, cinnamon and salt.
In another mixing bowl combine egg, juice and cooking oil.
Add flour to mixture all at once. Stir until just blended and ingredients are wet. (Batter should be a bit lumpy.) Fold in nuts.
Pour onto a lightly greased, hot griddle or skillet using an ¼ cup measure for regular size pancakes or 1 tablespoon measure for dollar size pancakes. Cook until pancakes are golden brown, turning to cook second side when pancakes have bubbly surfaces and dried edges.
Makes 8 standard-size pancakes or 36-dollar size pancakes.

Protein 2.8g
Iron 0.9mg

Raspberry Smoothie Bowl
From *realsimple.com*

Also, fulfills fruit, herb/spice, and whole grain requirements.

1 Raspberry Smoothie, recipe in the Beverage Recipes chapter.

Optional toppings:
1 kiwi, sliced
2 Tbsp. roasted almonds or walnuts, chopped
1 tsp. flaxseed or chia seeds
2 Tbsp. granola

Pour smoothie into bowl.
Top with above toppings. (Looks nice when toppings are placed in a line on top of the smoothie.)
Makes 2 servings.

Protein 9g
Iron 2.3mg

Roasted Pumpkin Seeds
From *Southern Lady*

Also, fulfills the herb/spice requirement.

6 c. raw shelled pumpkin seeds
¼ c. butter, melted
1 Tbsp. chili powder
1 Tbsp. ground cumin
1 tsp. garlic powder
1 tsp. salt
Coarse salt

Preheat oven to 250-degrees. Line roasting pan with aluminum foil. Place pumpkin seeds in large bowl.
In small bowl, combine melted butter, chili powder, cumin, garlic powder and salt, whisking to combine well. Pour butter mixture over pumpkin seeds; toss to coat. Spread pumpkin seeds in an even layer in prepared pan. Bake for 1 hour, stirring every 15 minutes.
Remove from oven and spread in single layer on parchment paper; sprinkle with coarse salt. Let cool completely.
Makes 6 cups. Store in air tight container and use by sprinkling on salads, soups and mashed or puréed vegetables. (Also, good as a snack source.)

Protein 9g, per cup of seeds
Iron 4.2mg, per cup of seeds

Roasted Stone-Fruit For 2
Adapted from *Real Simple* magazine

Also, fulfills fruit requirement.

¼ c. walnuts
1 Tbsp. unsalted butter
2 "stone fruit": nectarines, apricot, or plums, halved & pitted
1 tsp. sugar
3 oz. maple syrup
1 c. low-fat yogurt

Chop walnuts and place on a microwaveable dish. Cook at high-power 1-2 minutes. Stir and repeat if walnuts need more time to "toast." Set aside.
Melt butter in small cast-iron skillet on medium-high heat. Sprinkle plum halves evenly with sugar and place, cut-side down, in skillet. Cook until bottoms of plums are gold in color about 2-3 minutes. Turn plums **and reduce to medium heat;** cook an additional 5 or 6 minutes until tender. Remove plums to a small bowl. Leave pan on burner.
Add syrup to pan drippings and stir. Pour over plum halves. Note: Fruit and syrup can be refrigerated up to 2 days and be eaten cold or warmed.
To serve, divide yogurt into two bowls. Top with 2 halves of fruit and walnuts. Drizzle with syrup.
Makes 2 servings. (Also, makes a great dessert.)

Protein 12g
Iron 3.3mg

Sunflower Poppy Seed Muffins
Inspired by *Betty Crocker's New American Cooking*

Also, fulfills the herb/spice requirement.

1 egg
¾ c. almond milk
½ c. sunflower "nuts", lightly salted
1 Tbsp. poppy seeds
⅓ c. vegetable oil
¼ c. honey
2 c. whole wheat flour
3 tsp. baking powder
½ tsp. pumpkin pie spice

Preheat oven to 400-degrees. Grease bottom of muffin tin.
In large bowl, beat egg and stir in milk, seeds, oil and honey.
In separate, medium-size bowl, stir together flour, baking powder and salt. Add all of the dry ingredients to the egg mixture. Stir only until flour is incorporated. (Batter should be lumpy.)
Fill muffin cups ¾ full. (Sprinkle with granulated sugar if desired.) Bake until golden brown, about 15-20 minutes. Remove immediately from pan.
Makes 12; freeze leftovers in air-tight container.

Protein 5.1
Iron 1.4

Protein Recipes

BEEF ENTREES:
Baked Meatball Stew
Beef (Sa-tay) Satay

EGG ENTREES:
Baked Eggs in Bell Peppers
Vegetable Frittata with Greens

FISH ENTREES:
Pan-Fried Salmon Fillet for 2 with Dill Sauce
Tuna-Stuffed Peppers for Two

LEGUME ENTREES:
JP's Split Pea Soup
Mexican Black Bean Fusion

PORK ENTREES:
Confetti-Stuffed Pork Roast
Pork Tenderloin with Roasted Apples & Onions

POULTRY ENTREES:
Fiesta Turkey Soup
Nutty Beet & Chicken Salad with Maple Syrup Vinaigrette

Beef Entrees:

Baked Meatball Stew
Inspired by *Cooking Light*

Also, fulfills vegetable and herb/spice requirements.

1 lb. ground beef
½ c. soft breadcrumbs
2 Tbsp. Worcestershire sauce
½ tsp. garlic, minced
2 c. onion, chopped
2 c. russet potatoes, chopped
1 c. carrot, sliced
½ tsp. dried basil
¼ tsp. dried thyme
½ tsp. pepper
3 c. fat-free beef broth
1 ½ tsp. dried parsley

Combine meat, breadcrumbs, Worcestershire sauce, and garlic powder in medium bowl; stir well. Shape into meatballs, using about 1 tablespoon of mixture for each.
Place meatballs in large nonstick skillet, and cook over medium heat 8-10 minutes or until browned, turning frequently. Drain and pat dry with paper towels.
Arrange half of meatballs in 3-quart casserole. Layer half of onion, potato, and carrots over meatballs.
Combine basil, thyme, and pepper; sprinkle half of mixture over vegetables. Repeat.
Pour beef broth over layered vegetables. Cover and bake at 350-degrees for 1 hour and 15 minutes or until vegetables are tender.

Ladle stew into individual bowls and sprinkle with parsley. Makes 7 cups. (Freezes well.)

Protein 15g
Iron 2.2mg

Beef (Sa-Tay) Satay
Inspired by *Cooking Light*

Also, fulfills herb/spice requirement.

1 lb. lean round steak
⅓ c. lime juice
3 Tbsp. soy sauce
2 Tbsp. creamy, no salt peanut butter, melted
1 Tbsp. apple cider vinegar
1 tsp. chili powder
1 tsp. olive oil
Vegetable cooking spray
Garnish: Lime wedges

Partially freeze steak to make cutting easier.
Trim fat from steak and slice diagonally across grain into ¼-inch strips. Place strips in a large shallow dish. Add lime juice; cover and chill 4 hours. Whisk together soy sauce, peanut butter, vinegar, chili powder and oil until smooth. Set aside.
Place 12 6-inch wooden skewers in a basin of water to soak. Remove steak from marinade and thread on skewers. Coat rack of boiler pan with cooking spray. Place skewers on rack and broil 5 ½-inches from heat 2-3 minutes each side.
Arrange skewers on serving plate, garnish with lime wedges. Serve with small individual dishes of reserved soy sauce mixture.
Makes 12 skewers or 6 servings.

Protein 8.8g
Iron 2.5mg

Egg Entrees:

Baked Eggs In Bell Peppers
Inspired by *everydaypaleo.com*

Also, fulfills fruit (zucchini) and herb/spice requirements.

2 lg. red or yellow bell peppers, cut in half lengthwise and seeded. (Leave stem for a pretty finish.)
2 turkey sausage patties
½ c. zucchini, diced
½ c. yellow onion, diced
½ c. Portobello mushrooms, diced
2 cloves garlic, minced
4 lg. eggs
Sea salt, to taste
Black pepper, to taste

Garnish with fresh or dried basil
Preheat oven to 375 degrees.
Place bell pepper halves, cut side down, on lightly greased baking sheet and roast in oven 15-20 minutes.
Meanwhile fry sausage and set aside.
In the same pan, sauté the diced onion over medium to medium-high heat until it begins to soften. Add minced garlic, zucchini and mushrooms and sauté until zucchini are al dente. Crumble sausage and combine in sauté pan.
Once bell peppers are ready, dry inside of each pepper half with a paper towel and stuff with a large scoop of the sausage and veggie mixture. Press down with the back of a spoon to make an indentation for the egg mixture.
Whisk together eggs, salt and pepper. Pour evenly into the stuffed pepper halves.

Place stuffed bells in a large casserole dish, cover with foil and bake 30-40 minutes or until eggs are set; check after 20 minutes to determine final baking time.
Garnish with a sprinkle of chopped basil leaves.
Makes 4 servings.

Protein 9g
Iron 0.1mg

Vegetable Frittata With Greens
Adapted from *Real Simple* magazine

Also, fulfills fruit (tomatoes), and greens requirements.

1 Tbsp. olive oil
½ lb. asparagus, trimmed & cut into 1" pieces
1 c. frozen peas
½ c. cherry tomatoes
8 lg. eggs
1 tsp. salt
½ tsp. white pepper
2 oz. feta cheese, crumbled
1 tsp. white vinegar
1 ½ tsp. extra-virgin olive oil
3 c. assorted lettuce mixture

Preheat oven to 400-degrees F.
Place peas in microwaveable casserole. Add 1-2 tablespoons water and heat on high setting 6-7 minutes, stirring once.
Heat olive oil in nonstick, ovenproof skillet over medium-high heat. Add asparagus and cook 3 minutes until softened, stir occasionally.
Add microwaved peas and tomatoes to skillet. Cook about 5 more minutes until tomato skins burst, stir occasionally.
Whisk eggs, salt and pepper; pour mixture over vegetables in skillet. Cook, stirring gently, until eggs begin to set, about 1 minute. Sprinkle with cheese and transfer pan to oven. Bake 10-12 minutes until center is set.
While eggs are baking, mix together vinegar, extra-virgin olive oil with a pinch of salt and pepper. Toss with lettuce. Place on top of frittata. Cut and serve.
Makes 4-6 servings.

Protein 17g
Iron 3.3mg

Fish Entrees:

Pan-Fried Salmon Fillet For 2 With Dill Sauce
Adapted from *Real Simple* magazine

Also, fulfills herb/spice requirement.

1 6-oz. skin-on salmon fillet
1 Tbsp. olive oil

Heat oil in non-stick small skillet over medium-high heat. Add salmon, skin-side down. Cook 3-4 minutes or until fillet can be turned with skin. Cook until no longer translucent but moist in the center about 3-4 more minutes. Remove from skillet.
Let rest 5 minutes before serving or serve at room temperature. Cut fillet in half and serve.

SAUCE:
1/3 c. low-fat Greek yogurt
1 Tbsp. fresh lemon juice
1 tsp. fresh dill, chopped
¾ tsp. salt
¼ tsp. pepper

Mix sauce ingredients together. Place a tablespoon of sauce on top of salmon and serve.
Makes 2 servings of salmon with dill sauce.

Protein 19g
Iron 0.3mg

Tuna-Stuffed Peppers For Two
Adapted from *Prevention.com*

Also, fulfills herb/spice, vegetable and whole grain requirements.

½ c. quick-cooking barley
2 lg. red bell peppers, tops removed; seeded
Olive oil cooking spray
1 tsp. olive oil
1 5-oz. can solid white tuna, packed in water, drained
1 egg, beaten
⅛ c. grated Parmesan cheese
1 ½ Tbsp. finely chopped parsley (or ⅛ c. fresh parsley, finely chopped)
1 clove garlic, minced
½ sm. onion, minced
¼ tsp. dried Italian seasoning
⅛ tsp. black pepper
Salt, to taste
Garnish: parsley leaves, optional

Prepare barley according to package directions; set aside.
Preheat oven to 350-degrees. Spray baking pan with oil.
Bring 3 cups of water to a boil in large saucepan. Add peppers and reduce heat to simmer. Cook 5 minutes.
Place peppers in colander; run under cold water to stop cooking process. Dry peppers and then rub with olive oil and place in baking pan.
In bowl, stir together barley, tuna, egg, cheese, parsley, garlic, onion, and seasonings until well blended. Place half of mixture in each bell pepper. Bake 40 minutes.
Season with salt if desired. Garnish with fresh Italian parsley leaf.
Makes 2 servings.

Protein 14g
Iron 2.3mg

Legume Entrees:

Jp's Split Pea Soup
From John Pizza

Also, fulfills vegetable requirement.

1 16-oz. pkg. split-peas, rinsed & drained
1 med. onion, diced
1 Tbsp. olive oil
1 Tbsp. bacon grease
5 c. water
1 Tbsp. ham base
1 c. milk
Garnish: Croutons

Heat oil in large sauce pan or Dutch oven on medium-high; add onions and sauté until translucent; add peas and sauté lightly.
Add water and bring to boiling. Lower heat and simmer 60-90 minutes, stirring occasionally until peas are soft. Turn off heat, leaving pan on burner.
Stir in ham base. Use submersible blender or hand mixer to break peas down into a light purée, add milk; stir and heat through.
Ladle into shallow soup bowls; garnish with croutons.
Makes 8 servings. Freezes well.

Protein 15g
Iron 2.5mg

Mexican Black Bean Fusion

Inspired by *Cooking Light Cookbook*

Fulfills protein, fruit (tomato), herb/spice and whole grain requirements.

2 tsp. olive oil
½ white onion, chopped
¼ c. green pepper, chopped
1 c. cooked couscous
¼ tsp. cumin
⅛ tsp. paprika
Pinch of dried coriander
1 c. black beans, rinsed & drained
½ c. cherry tomatoes, chopped
Optional: lime, cut into wedges

Heat oil in large nonstick skillet over medium-high heat until hot. Add onions and green pepper; sauté until tender.
Stir in couscous, cumin, paprika, and coriander; sauté 3 minutes. Add beans and cherry tomatoes, sauté an additional 3 minutes or until heated through.
Serve with lime wedges for additional flavoring, if desired.
Makes 4 servings.

Protein 3.8g
Iron 1.4mg

Pork Entrees:

Confetti-Stuffed Pork Roast
Adapted from *Cooking Light Cookbook*

Also, fulfills fruit (zucchini), herb/spice and vegetable requirements.

Olive oil cooking spray
½ c. carrot, shredded
½ c. zucchini, shredded
½ c. sweet red pepper, diced
¼ c. onion, finely chopped
2 tsp. dried parsley
2 Tbsp. white wine vinegar
2 ½ lb. lean boneless double pork loin roast
½ tsp. dried basil
¼ tsp. dried thyme
¼ tsp. pepper

Garnish: fresh basil springs
Coat medium nonstick skillet with cooking spray and place over medium-high heat until hot. Add carrot, zucchini, red pepper and onion; sauté until tender. Stir in parsley and vinegar. Cook, uncovered, until liquid is absorbed.
Trim fat on roast and butterfly. Spread vegetable mixture over inside of roast. With cooking twine, tie roast in four places.
Combine basil, thyme, and pepper; rub over surface of roast. Coat roasting pan and rack with cooking spray. Place roast on top of rack and bake, uncovered at 325-degrees for 2 hours or until meat thermometer registers 170-degrees. Let roast stand 10 minutes.

Remove string and slice roast diagonally across grain into ¼-inch thick slices; arrange on large serving platter. If desired, garnish with fresh basil sprigs for a pretty presentation.
Makes 10 servings. (Freezes well.)

Protein 26g
Iron 1.0mg

Pork Tenderloin With Roasted Apples & Onions
Adapted from *catholicdigest.com*

Also, fulfills fruit and herb/spice requirements.

1 10-oz. pork tenderloin
Salt and pepper, to taste
3 Tbsp. olive oil, divided
2 Tbsp. Dijon mustard
1 lg. onion, sliced
2 med. Granny Smith apples, peeled, cored & sliced ¼-inch thick
½ c. apple juice

Preheat oven to 450-degrees. Season pork with salt and pepper.
Heat 2 tablespoons oil in large nonstick, ovenproof skillet over medium-high heat. Add pork and sear until all sides are brown, turning occasionally, about 5 minutes.
Transfer pork to plate. Cool slightly. Spread mustard over top and side of pork.
Add remaining oil to skillet. Sauté onion slices and apples over medium heat until golden, about 5 minutes. Spread evenly in skillet and sprinkle with salt and pepper. Place pork on top of apple-onion mixture.
Transfer skillet to oven and roast until apple-onion mixture is soft and brown. Center of pork should register 160-degrees on meat thermometer, about 15-20 minutes.
Transfer pork to dish and tent with foil. Let stand 5 minutes.
Meanwhile pour apple juice over apple-onion mixture in skillet. Stir mixture over high heat until slightly reduced, about 2 minutes.
Cut pork diagonally into ½-inch thick slices. Spoon apple-onion mixture onto platter. Top with pork and serve.
Makes 4 servings.

Protein 21g
Iron 1.2mg

Poultry Entrees:

Fiesta Turkey Soup
Adapted from *Eat for Extraordinary Health Cookbook*

Also, fulfills herb/spice and vegetable requirements.

1 Tbsp. olive oil
1 sm. onion, chopped
1 sm. jalapeño pepper
1 med. zucchini chopped
2 tsp. ground cumin
½ tsp. ancho chili powder
1 lb. 99% fat-free ground turkey
1 carton 32-oz. low-sodium chicken broth
1 14.5-oz. can diced tomatoes
1 15-oz. can black beans, rinsed and drained
1 c. frozen corn kernels
½ c. fresh cilantro, chopped
½ c. avocado, chopped
6 Tbsp. Cheddar cheese, shredded

Wearing plastic gloves, seed and finely chop pepper.

In large saucepan, heat oil over medium-high heat. Cook onion and pepper, stirring occasionally, for 5 minutes or until lightly browned. Stir in zucchini, cumin, and chili powder. Cook 10 minutes or until zucchini is lightly browned.
Add turkey and cook, stirring to break up turkey for 5 minutes or until no longer pink.
Stir in broth, tomatoes with juice, beans and corn. Bring to a boil over high heat. Lower heat and simmer 20 minutes or until liquid is reduced by one-quarter. Remove from heat. Stir in cilantro. Divide

among six bowls. Sprinkle each serving with a spoonful of avocado and a tablespoon of cheese.
Makes 6 servings.

Protein 22g
Iron 1.5mg

Nutty Beet & Chicken Salad With Maple Syrup Vinaigrette

Also, fulfills greens, vegetable and nut/seed requirements.

1 can sliced red beets
¼ c. candied pecans – see below
¼ c. feta cheese, crumbled
1 c. cooked chicken, cut into small bite-size pieces
½ c. spinach leaves
1 Tbsp. maple syrup
2 Tbsp. vinegar
1 Tbsp. olive oil

Combine beets, pecans, cheese, and chicken. Line salad dishes with spinach leaves. Place combined ingredients on top of leaves.
Prepare vinaigrette by whisking together the maple syrup, vinegar and oil. Serve over top of salad.
Serves 2.

CANDIED PECANS:
1 egg white
2 tsp. water
¼ c. sugar
½ tsp. cinnamon
¼ c. whole pecans

Preheat oven to 250-degrees. Whisk egg white and water until frothy. In separate bowl, combine sugar and cinnamon.

Place pecans in egg white; remove and toss in the cinnamon sugar mixture. Spread coated pecans on baking sheet and bake 1 hour, stirring every 15 minutes, until evenly browned.

Protein 37g
Iron 3.0mg

Vegetable Recipes

B. J.'s Simple Sautéed Carrots
Blue Cheese Asparagus
Classic Succotash
Corn & Black Bean Salsa Salad
Country Baked Lime Bean Casserole
Gruyère Onions
Peas & Noodles Parmigiano
Potato Hash with Okra
Sautéed Pepper Quesadillas
Tomato-Potato-Zucchini Tian

B. J.'S Simple Sautéed Carrots
From B. J. Byars for *ENJOY! Recipes for Fresh Produce*

Also, fulfills the herb/spice requirement.

Carrots with green tops if possible
Butter
Cinnamon

Clean and peel carrots, cut lengthwise. (Pretty when about 1-inch of green tops are left on carrots.)
Fry with a little butter in sauté pan on medium-high heat, sprinkle with cinnamon.
Simple, elegant, & tasty! It doesn't get easier.

1 medium carrot equals 0.7g Protein and 0.4mg Iron.

Blue Cheese Asparagus
Adapted from *Cooking Light Cookbook*

Also, fulfills nut/seed requirement.

2 Tbsp. pecans, chopped
1 ½ lb. asparagus spears
Vegetable cooking spray
2 tsp. butter
2 Tbsp. cider vinegar
3 Tbsp. feta cheese, crumbled

In large non-stick fry pan, toast pecans, stirring until fragrant.
Snap off tough ends of asparagus; remove hard scales.
Coat pan with cooking spray, add butter. Place over medium heat until butter melts.
Add asparagus and sauté 3-4 minutes. Add vinegar, cover and simmer 2-3 minutes or until asparagus is crisp-tender.
Add cheese and pecans; toss gently.
Serve warm.
Makes 6 servings.

Protein 3
Iron 0.6

Classic Succotash
Adapted from *southernliving.com*

Also, fulfills the fruit (tomatoes) and herb/spice requirements.

1 c. fresh lima beans
¼ sm. yellow onion
2 sprigs fresh thyme
½ clove garlic
1 ½ slices bacon
½ med. sweet onion, chopped
3 ears corn, kernels cut from cobs
½ pt. cherry tomatoes, halved
1 Tbsp. butter
1 ½ tsp. red wine vinegar
1 ¾ tsp. fresh dill, chopped
1 ¾ tsp. fresh chives, chopped

Place beans, onion, thyme and garlic in saucepan, cover with water and bring to a boil over medium-high heat. Reduce heat to medium and simmer, stirring occasionally, 20 minutes or until beans are tender. Drain beans, reserving ½ cup cooking liquid. Discard onion, thyme and garlic.
Cook bacon in medium-size skillet over medium heat 7 minutes or until crisp, turning once. Remove bacon, reserving 1 tablespoon drippings in skillet. Drain bacon on paper towels and crumble.
Sauté chopped sweet onion in hot drippings over medium-high heat for 5 minutes. Stir in corn and cook, stirring often about 6 minutes or until corn is tender. Stir tomatoes, cooked beans and reserved cooking liquid into pan. Cook, stirring occasionally, 5 minutes.
Stir butter, vinegar, dill and chives into pan.
Season with salt and pepper. Sprinkle with crumbled bacon.
Makes 2 large servings.

Protein 8g
Iron 1.6mg

Corn & Black Bean Salsa Salad
From *ENJOY! Recipes for Fresh Produce*

Also, fulfills the greens, herb/spice, protein requirements.

SALAD:
1 15-oz. can black beans, rinsed & drained
2 ears corn, cooked & cut from cob
1 red sweet pepper, cut into ½-inch pieces
1 stalk celery, sliced
1 Tbsp. cilantro, snipped
Lettuce leaves for salad bowls
Garnish: avocado slices

DRESSING:
¼ c. plain Greek yogurt
¼ c. mayonnaise
¼ c. salsa
¼ tsp. cumin

In large bowl combine salad ingredients except lettuce and avocado.
In a screw-top jar, combine dressing ingredients and shake.
Add dressing to salad and toss. Cover and chill 2-24 hours.
Line salad bowls with lettuce leaves and garnish with avocado slices.
Makes 6 servings.

Protein 7g
Iron 1.7mg

Country Baked Lime Bean Casserole
Adapted from *Betty Crocker's New American Cooking*

Also, fulfills the herb/spice, and protein requirements.

½ lb. dried lima beans, rinse & drain
2 c. water
½ large sweet onion, sliced
2 slices bacon, chopped
½ c. tomato juice
¼ c. honey
2 Tbsp. chili sauce
½ tsp. salt
½ tsp. prepared yellow mustard

Place beans in 2-quart sauce pan, cover with water. Bring to boiling and cook 1-2 minutes; cover and remove from heat. Rest for 1 hour.
If necessary, add water to just cover beans. Heat to boiling and then reduce heat to simmer, uncovered, for 30 minutes. (Bean skins should not split, so make sure beans do not boil.)
After final simmer, reserve liquid and drain beans. Preheat oven to 300-degrees.
In lightly greased 2-quart casserole, layer beans, onions and bacon.
Mix tomato juice, honey, chili sauce, salt and mustard and pour over beans. Add only enough reserved liquid to cover.
Cover and cook one hour; stir.
Uncover and cook an additional 30 minutes.
Makes 6, half-cup servings.

Protein 14g
Iron 3.8mg

Gruyère Onions

From *ENJOY! Recipes for Fresh Produce*

Also, fulfills the herb/spice requirements.

2 ½ med. Vidalia onions
1 tsp. olive oil
Salt, to taste
Pepper, to taste
½ cube beef bouillon
½ c. water
1 tsp. low-sodium soy sauce
2 oz. Gruyère smoked cheese, finely shredded
1 tsp. sage, minced

Preheat oven to 400-degrees. Coat shallow baking dish, large enough to hold 5 onion halves, with cooking spray.
Trim 1/4-inch off top and bottom of onions; cut onions in half cross-wise, and peel. Arrange, cut sides up, in baking dish.
Brush tops of each half onion with oil and sprinkle with salt and pepper. Bake 35 minutes.
Boil water, dissolve bouillon cube. Mix broth with soy sauce. Pour over onions and continue baking 1 hour; baste occasionally. Add water, if necessary.
Sprinkle each onion half evenly with cheese and sage. Bake 5-7 minutes more.
Makes 5 halves; can easily be doubled.

Protein 9g
Iron 0mg

Peas & Noodles Parmigiano
Adapted from *ENJOY! Recipes for Fresh Produce*

8 oz. egg noodles, prepared with 1 tsp. salt, drained
1 tsp. salt
2 Tbsp. olive oil
2 med. scallions, sliced ⅛" thick lengthwise
2 c. frozen green peas, shelled
1-2 Tbsp. grated (Parmigiana) Italian Cheese mixture
½ tsp. pepper

Heat oil in large frying or sauté pan over medium-high heat until barely smoking. Add scallions and peas. Sauté for 5-7 minutes, stirring frequently. Remove from heat.
Test peas by slightly mashing with back of spoon, when "mashable", continue mashing half of the peas.
Add noodles to pan, place on medium heat, stir and heat through.
When ready to serve place in serving dish and garnish with cheese and pepper.
Makes 4-6 servings.

Protein 5g
Iron 1.0mg

Potato Hash With Okra

From *ENJOY! Recipes for Fresh Produce*

Also, fulfills the nut & seed and herb/spice requirements.

1 Tbsp. whole mustard seeds
⅓ c. olive oil
½ clove garlic, minced
1 sm. Vidalia onion, diced small
2 tsp. ginger, minced
½ lb. russet potatoes, diced small
½ tsp. red pepper flakes
½ tsp. salt
¼ tsp. pepper
1 ½ lb. okra, cut into ⅛" rounds
2 tsp. ground cumin
2 tsp. ground coriander
1 tsp. ground turmeric
1 ½ Tbsp. salted toasted sesame seeds

Heat oil in large heavy skillet or wok on medium-high, add mustard seeds and heat 10 seconds or until seeds begin to pop.
Add onion, garlic and ginger to pan and sauté until fragrant, about 2 minutes.
Stir in potatoes, red pepper flakes, salt and pepper. Cover pan and reduce heat to low. Cook, stirring occasionally, 5 minutes.
Uncover and stir in okra and rest of spices. Cook, stirring occasionally, 8-10 minutes until potatoes and okra are tender. Salt and pepper to taste. Just before serving, sprinkle with sesame seeds.
Makes 4-6 servings.

Protein 6.7g
Iron 2.2mg

Sautéed Pepper Quesadillas
Adapted from *foodheavenmadeeasy.com*

Also, fulfills protein requirement.

1 bell pepper
½ c. mushrooms
¼ c. onion
1 Tbsp. oil
¼ tsp. salt
4 flour tortillas
2 oz. hard cheese, shredded

Slice pepper into strips; slice mushrooms and onions.
Heat sauté pan on medium and add oil. Add vegetables and sauté 4-5 minutes. Salt and remove from pan.
Place one tortilla in same pan and brown on one side; set aside. Place a second tortilla in pan and layer with half of the pepper mixture and top with the prepared tortilla. Cook until bottom tortilla is crisp and cheese has melted, about 2 minutes. Cut into quarters.
Repeat process with the remaining tortillas.
Makes 4 servings.

Protein 2.0g
Iron 4.4mg

Tomato-Potato-Zucchini Tian

From *ENJOY! Recipes for Fresh Produce*

Also, fulfills protein (cheese) requirements.

Olive oil cooking spray
3 Tbsp. butter, divided
1 med. Vidalia onion, chopped
2 med. Yukon gold potatoes, sliced very thin
1 med. zucchini, sliced ¼" thick
4 plum tomatoes, sliced ¼" thick
1 ½ tsp. salt
¾ tsp. black pepper
1 ⅓ c. Parmesan cheese, grated

Preheat oven to 375-degrees. Spray to coat 8-inch quiche dish or casserole. Melt 2 tablespoons butter in medium pan over medium heat; add onions, and sauté about 10 minutes until nearly caramelized. Turn off heat.
Spoon onions into dish. Place remaining butter in hot pan and let melt. Toss together sliced vegetables with salt and pepper. Arrange in dish alternately, overlapping slightly, in a single layer over onions; drizzle with the butter from the pan.
Cover dish and bake 30 minutes.
Uncover, sprinkle with cheese, and bake another 35-40 minutes. Let stand 10 minutes before serving.
May be served hot or warm.
Makes 6 servings.

Protein 19g
Iron 1.5mg

Whole Grain Recipes

Banana-Oat Bran Pancakes
Barley & Vegetables
Carrot-Wild Rice Stuffing
Diana's Protein Bars
Green Pea Pesto Toasts with Soft-Cooked Eggs
Overnight Oats with Fruit
Rice & Walnuts
Super Yummy Grilled Sandwich
Tropical Oatmeal
Wild Rice Pancakes

Banana-Oat Bran Pancakes

Adapted from *Cooking Light Cookbook*

Also, fulfills fruit and protein requirements.

¾ c. unprocessed oat bran
¾ c. all-purpose flour
1 tsp. baking powder
1 tsp. baking soda
1 Tbsp. sugar
1 8-oz. carton plain low-fat yogurt
½ c. mashed ripe banana
1 Tbsp. vegetable oil
2 tsp. vanilla extract
3 eggs
Vegetable cooking spray

Combine oat bran, flour, baking powder, baking soda, and sugar in medium bowl; make a well in the center of dry ingredients.

Combine yogurt, banana, oil, vanilla and eggs; pour into the well in the dry ingredients, stirring until moistened.

For each pancake, pour ¼ cup batter onto hot griddle or skillet coated with cooking spray. Turn pancakes when tops are covered with broken bubbles and edges appear dry.

Makes 12 4-inch pancakes or 4 servings of 3 each.

[Delicious with Strawberry Sauce which can be found in the Fruit Recipes chapter.]

Protein 8g
Iron 1.1mg

Barley & Vegetables
Adapted from *Betty Crocker's New American Cooking*

Also, fulfills fruit (zucchini), and herb/spice requirements.

3 c. water
1 c. uncooked barley
1 Tbsp. instant beef bouillon
2 sm. zucchini, cut into ½-inch slices
2 med. stalks celery, sliced
1 sm. onion, chopped
1 c. mushrooms, sliced
¾ tsp. dried basil leaves
2 Tbsp. butter
1 2-oz. jar diced pimiento, drained
½ tsp. salt
1 Tbsp. lemon juice

Heat water, barley and bouillon to boiling in 3-quart saucepan; reduce heat. Cover and simmer until barley is tender and liquid is absorbed, about 1 hour.
Cook and stir zucchini, celery, onion, mushrooms and basil in butter in 10-inch skillet until celery is crisp-tender, about 10 minutes.
Stir barley, pimiento and salt into pan. Cover over medium heat, stirring occasionally, until barley is hot, about 5 minutes.
Stir in lemon juice and serve.
Makes 8 servings.

Protein 4g
Iron 0.4mg

Carrot-Wild Rice Stuffing
Adapted from *Cooking Light Cookbook*

Also, fulfills fruit, vegetable and herb/spice requirements.

1 ½ c. cooked wild rice
⅔ c. apple, chopped
⅔ c. green onions, sliced
⅔ c. carrot, shredded
¼ c. + 3 Tbsp. water
2 Tbsp. almonds, chopped & toasted
2 Tbsp. golden raisins
2 Tbsp. lemon juice
1 Tbsp. butter
¼ tsp. cinnamon
¼ tsp. nutmeg
¼ tsp. salt
¼ tsp. pepper

(If you haven't already done so, cook wild rice according to package directions. Keep warm.)
Combine apple, onions, carrot, water, almonds and raisins; place in a 2-quart casserole, stir well and mist with water. Add rest of ingredients; stir well. Cover and microwave on high 5 minutes; stirring after 2 minutes. Remove when mixture boils.
Reduce heat to low (10% power) and microwave an additional 2 minutes. Remove from microwave, add rice; adjust cover to allow steam to escape and let stand 10 minutes
Stir well and serve.
Makes 4 servings.

Protein 3g
Iron 0.8mg

Diana's Protein Bars
From Diana Hale

Also, fulfills protein requirement.

2 c. whole oats
2 c. peanut butter
¼ c. honey
⅓ c. semi-sweet or dark chocolate chips

Preheat oven to 350-degrees.
In large bowl, mix together oats, peanut butter, and honey until well combined.
Spread mixture in a 13 x 9" baking pan or rimmed cookie sheet.
Sprinkle chocolate chips evenly over top. Bake 10 minutes.
Remove from heat and using an icing knife, spread chips over bars. (Chips will melt to make an icing-like topping.) Cool for 5 minutes.
Cut into 12 large bars. Place cooled pan of bars in refrigerator to solidify completely. Remove bars from pan; store in an airtight container in refrigerator.

Makes 12 bars.
Protein 11.3g
Iron 0.9mg

Green Pea Pesto Toasts With Soft-Cooked Eggs
From *Martha Stewart magazine*

Also, fulfills protein, nut & seed and herb/spice requirements.

½ c. fresh or frozen green peas
½ c. basil leaves
½ c. extra-virgin olive oil
Pinch of salt
3 cloves
½ c. Parmesan cheese
¼ c. walnuts, finely chopped
2 soft-boiled eggs, sliced in half
4 lg. whole wheat crackers

Purée peas in food processor, add basil, walnuts, garlic, cheese, and oil to make a spread.
Place spread on toasts or crackers. Top with egg.
Makes 2 servings.
[Spread also makes an easy sauce for pasta.]

Protein 30g
Iron 2.4mg

Overnight Oats With Fruit
Adapted from *Better Homes and Gardens*

Also, fulfills fruit (berry), herb/spice and nuts & seed requirements.

2 c. regular rolled oats
1 c. almond milk
1 c. apple juice
¼ c. honey
1 tsp. cinnamon
¾ c. blanched almonds, pecans, or walnuts – toasted & coarsely chopped
1 tart green apple, cored, seeded, sliced thinly & chopped
1 6-oz. container low-fat plain yogurt
1 c. fresh or thawed frozen raspberries

Place ½ cup oats in four ½-pint (8 ounce) jars or containers.
In a large pitcher (or a 4-cup measure) combine milk, apple juice, honey and cinnamon. Pour over oats in jars. Cover; chill overnight or until oats are soft.
Stir in nuts and top with yogurt, apple and raspberries. Serve with extra honey for sweet lovers.
Makes 4 servings.

Protein 17g
Iron 3.6mg

Rice & Walnuts

Inspired by *Betty Crocker's New American Cooking*

Also, fulfills fruit, and herb/spice requirements.

½ c. quick-cooking brown rice
½ med. onion, chopped
1 clove garlic, minced
1 Tbsp. olive oil
1 ¼ c. water
¼ c. raisins
1½ tsp. chicken bouillon
¼ tsp. dry mustard
Pinch of pepper
1 oz. walnuts, toasted & chopped
⅛ c. fresh Italian Parsley, snipped

Cook rice according to package direction.
Place oil in 1-quart saucepan over medium heat; add onion and garlic and cook until onion is tender, about 5 minutes.
Stir in water, raisins, bouillon, mustard and pepper; heat to boiling. Reduce heat to simmer and cover. Add rice and stir in nuts and parsley. Makes 4 servings. [Can easily be packed into cooking "rounds" for a pleasing presentation on the plate.]

Protein 4g
Iron 0.7mg

Super Yummy Grilled Sandwich

Also, fulfills fruit and possibly nut/seed (if nut spread is used) requirements.

4 slices whole wheat bread [Try, Eureka Saaa-Wheat bread.]
2 Tbsp. coconut oil
1 med. apple, cored & thinly sliced (save 2 pieces for garnish)
4 Tbsp. almond butter, walnut butter, plain butter, peanut butter or any nut spread

Spread coconut oil on one side of each slice of bread. Spread butter or nut spread on the other side of each slice.
Place half of the apple slices in between two slices of bread, coconut oil side out. Repeat with other two slices.
In medium skillet, on low heat, toast sandwiches until lightly brown, like a grilled-cheese sandwich.
Garnish with a piece of apple, skewered on a toothpick and placed in the top of each sandwich.
Makes 2

Protein 3.6g
Iron 1.2mg

Tropical Oatmeal
Adapted from *Foodheavenmadeeasy.com*

Fulfills protein, fruit, and herb/spice requirements.

½ c. oatmeal
1 Tbsp. peanut butter
½ banana, mashed
¼ to ½ tsp. cinnamon
1-2 tsp. honey

Prepare oatmeal and mix together with the peanut butter and banana. Sprinkle with cinnamon.
Makes two ¾ cup servings; can easily be doubled.

Protein 10g
Iron 1.8mg

Wild Rice Pancakes

Adapted from *Cooking Light Cookbook*

Also, fulfills protein requirements.

1 ¼ c. all-purpose flour
1 tsp. baking powder
½ tsp. baking soda
¼ tsp. salt
1 tsp. sugar
1 ¼ c. almond milk
2 eggs, separated, at room temperature
1 c. wild rice, cooked
2 Tbsp. butter, melted
3 egg whites, at room temperature
Coconut oil for pan

Combine flour, baking powder, baking soda, salt, and sugar in medium bowl; make a well in center.
In another bowl combine buttermilk and 2 egg yolks; add to dry ingredients, stirring just until moistened. Stir in wild rice and melted butter.
With electric mixer, on high speed, beat 5 egg whites in large bowl until stiff peaks form. Gently fold egg whites into batter.
Melt 1 teaspoon coconut oil in hot griddle or skillet. For each pancake, pour ¼ cup batter onto griddle or pan. Turn pancakes when tops are covered with broken bubbles and edges appear dry.
Makes 20 4-inch pancakes, or 4 servings of 5 pancakes each.

Protein 15g
Iron 3.5mg

Planning to Use The Plan

The first sentence of this book's introduction is, "Failure to plan is one reason why many people tend to not eat better." So, here are some planning tips.

Write out a weekly menu including your meals and snacks. Eventually you will settle on a few standby items to have for breakfast and snacks, but in the beginning this is the best way to begin using the Eat to Breathe Plan.

After dinner, the night before, place frozen food into the refrigerator; place other food items nearby. These will be visual reminders so the next morning, you'll remember what you planned for breakfast, what you're planning to eat for your other meals and any prep you need to do for that day.

If you begin to feel full and uncomfortable with the amount of food you are eating, reduce the serving size slightly but not the food group.

To save yourself money and prep time, make food ahead and put in serving size containers, if possible.

Always have a lot of good snacks available. Place nuts, granola, raisins, etc., in small, closable baggies and throw a few in your car or purse so when you get delayed and it's snack time, you've got something to eat and you won't be tempted to have that candy bar!

But, if you "cave-in" and eat that candy bar or piece of cake, don't beat yourself up. This isn't a weight-loss diet plan; it's a plan to better living. Just remember the goal, which is to breathe and live better, and you shouldn't have any problems staying on the plan.

Your Toolbox

My biggest hurdle in learning to live with COPD was accepting that it was now part of me and would be with me for the rest of my life. So how do we live the best life possible with it?

The eating plan I've provided is a start and as I say, one important tool in our tool box. What are the other tools?

▪ Tool #1: Quit Smoking

If you haven't quit smoking, there's no point in reading further. There's no point in working the plan. There's no point in putting any of these tools to use. *You simply must quit smoking.*

Quitting is hard, but it is what needs to be done to better your well-being. Talk to your doctor and get help: a patch, a pill, a group or a buddy. Just do it!

It took me multiple tries to quit smoking. I tried everything including acupuncture/hypnosis. I tried Chantix® not once but 3 times. The last time, when I decided to follow the directions exactly and see it through, I succeeded. You can do it. You must do it!

- ## Tool #2: Exercise

I'm going to use that nasty word again so cover your ears, "Exercise!" I know, I hate that word too but it is crucial to feeling the best you can while living with COPD. Begin low and slow by just walking. Walk with your oxygen if you must, but walk. Go to the mall; use a cart if necessary. Go online and find some recommended COPD exercises and breathing techniques. Ask your doctor to get you on the list for pulmonary rehab. These rehab professionals can help you safely know what exercise works best for you. Keeping muscles strong and oxygenated only happens with exercise. To quote my husband, "If it was fun, it would be called, fun-out not work-out!"

- ## Tool #3: Tweak Your Lifestyle

Most odors are not your friends. Gradually get rid of aerosols or sprays such as hair spray, perfume or deodorants. Do not use plug-in air fresheners or scented candles. Purchase pump sprays and roll-on deodorants. Instead of scented candles, try growing lavender plants in a sunny window. To add a healthy fragrance to your home, brew some cinnamon "tea".

Remove toxic cleaners that have fumes such as bleach, ammonia, bug and garden sprays.

Use vinegar, baking soda and borax or peroxide to clean.

Avoid dust and dirt. Use a N-95 dust mask when shaking out rugs, vacuuming or sweeping. Miracle cloths are wonderful, they trap dust and dirt and are reusable after washing. Also, change your vacuum, dryer and furnace filters often. Clean your refrigerator coils. Have your heating vents cleaned.

Avoid using fireplaces.

Bacteria, mold and mildew are on the no-no list. Replace sponges often or clean them in the dishwasher. Seal water leaks to avoid mold and mildew. Watch indoor humidity levels with a meter and try to keep it below 40 percent.

Pay attention to outside conditions. Air pollution can affect everyone but is especially bad for people with lung disease. Stay indoors and keep your windows closed on days when there is a high level of pollution. The local news station usually reports each day's pollution level. "Avoid breathing in bad fumes when traveling by car by avoiding rush hour times," suggests the COPD Foundation literature.

▪ Tool #4: Call in The Professionals

When things get beyond the control of our toolbox, we need to call in the professionals! Look at it this way: you are now the CEO of your body and you will need to use specialists to make your body the best it can be. So, get the best team of professionals on your side.

Find a GP (general practitioner). Have your yearly well-patient visits and labs each year. Get a referral to a qualified pulmonologist (lung doctor).

Your pulmonologist and you will begin to examine and build your specific formula to better living. Visit as frequently as your insurance company will allow. The more you two talk, the quicker you can get on the path to good health.

These two professionals will help you tap into a network of other individuals, i.e., respiratory specialists, physical rehabilitation therapists and nutritionists. With these people on your team, you can add quality years to your life!

- **Tool #5: Stay Current**

Make sure you get your wellness visit every six months with your General Practitioner. Stay up-to-date on immunizations. Visit your pulmonologist every six months and have your monitoring tests done on time.

- **Tool #6: Keep Up-To-Date**

You've taken the first step by buying this book. When you begin to use this plan, you will have taken the next step. Utilizing the other tools listed will help you gain energy and confidence.

Lastly, find ways to keep up-to-date with therapies, medications, and procedures. Ask your doctor for support groups or go on-line. Don't be an ostrich by hiding your head in the sand. As CEO of your body, your job is to know all you can so you can control your COPD and not let it control you!

Sources

AARP The Magazine/Real Possibilities
ADA – American Diabetes Association
AHA – American Heart Association
AND – Academy of Nutrition & Dietetics
Chef Grant Alford
Ancestralchef.com
BHG.com
The Baby Cookbook via Nytegiori
Better Homes and Gardens magazine
Better Homes and Gardens New Cook Book
Betty Crocker's New American Cooking
B. J. Byars
COPD Digest. Vol. 12, Number 2
caring.com
catholicdigest.com
Cleveland Clinic
Cooking Light Cookbook
Cooking with Curtis
countryliving.com
Eat for Extraordinary Health Cookbook
ENJOY! Recipes for Fresh Produce
European Respiratory Journal/nitrates/COPD
everydayhealth.com

everydaypaleo.com
foodheavenmadeeasy.com
The Global Burden of Disease Study
Michael Greger, M.D.
Diana Hale
Harvard T. H. Chan School of Public Health
health.com
Health & Healing
Healthline Networks, Inc.
Health Monitor/Guide to Living with COPD
Healthy Eating.org
How Not to Die
Light & Luscious
Martha Stewart magazine
Mary Miller
National Center for Health
nutritionaction.com
nutritionfacts.org
Emmett Oz, M.D.
John Pizza
lunginstitute.com
prevention.com
RD.com
Real Simple magazine
realsimple.com
Chef Kacy Rothwell, Wild Plum Tea Room, Gatlinburg, TN
Scripps Networks
The StayWell Company, LLC
Southern Lady magazine
Southern Living magazine
southernliving.com
USDA Department of Agriculture
uwhealth.org
University of Wisconsin Health Department

The View from Great Island.com blog
Connie Walker
WEBmd.com
White Westinghouse Microwave Oven Cookbook

Support Organizations and Resources Not Listed Elsewhere

www.aacvpr.org
www.aafa.org
www.alpha-1foundation.org
www.cff.org
www.coalitionforpf.org
www.copd-alert.com
www.copdcouncil.org
www.copdfoundation.org
copd-international.com
www.copd-support.com
www.emphysema.net
www.homeoxygen.org
www.LearnAboutCOPD.org
www.lung.org
www.nlhelp.org
www.nhlbi.nih.gov
www.nlhep.org
www.perf2ndwind.org
www.pulmonarypaper.org

www.smokefree.gov
www.uscopdcoalition.org
www.webmd.com/lung/copd
www.wellspouse.org

Recipe Index

APPLE & FENNEL SALAD	48	CORN & BLACK BEAN SALSA SALAD	95
ARUGULA WITH PLUM SAUCE	36	COUNTRY BAKED LIME BEAN CASSEROLE	96
B. J.'s SIMPLE SAUTÉED CARROTS	92	COUSCOUS FRUIT & VEGETABLE SALAD	61
BAKED EGGS IN BELL PEPPERS	76	DIANA'S PROTEIN BARS	107
BAKED MEATBALL STEW	73	ENGLISH WASSAIL	25
BAKED VEGETABLE OMELET	37	FARRO SALAD WITH TOASTED PECANS	62
BANANA NUT SALAD	60	FIESTA TURKEY SOUP	86
BANANA-BERRY SMOOTHIE	24	FRESH LEMONADE OR LIMEADE	26
BANANA-OAT BRAN PANCAKES	104	FRUIT SALAD WITH LIME	50
BARLEY & VEGETABLES	105	FRUIT SALAD WITH PEANUT BUTTER DRESSING	39
BEEF (SA-TAY) SATAY	75	GERMAN CHOCOLATE CAFÉ AU LAIT	27
BEET GREENS SIDE DISH	38	GRANNY'S RADICCHIO, APPLE & CELERY ROOT SALAD	40
BLUE CHEESE ASPARAGUS	93		
CARROT-WILD RICE STUFFING	106		
CINNAMON-APPLE OATMEAL	49		
CLASSIC SUCCOTASH	94	GREEN PEA PESTO TOASTS WITH SOFT-COOKED EGGS	108
CONFETTI-STUFFED PORK ROAST	83		

GRUYÈRE ONIONS	97	SAUTÉED PEPPER	
JP'S SPLIT PEA SOUP	81	QUESADILLAS	100
KALE & QUINOA SALAD	41	SIMPLE PAPAYA AVOCADO	
KIWI BANANA SHAKE for 2	28	SALAD	54
MARY'S ROASTED PEAR SALAD	64	SPINACH CARROT SALAD	43
MEXICAN BLACK BEAN		SPINACH TACOS	44
FUSION	82	SPRING GREEN & BEAN	
MULLED WINE	29	SALAD	45
NUTTY BEET & CHICKEN		STRAWBERRY SAUCE	55
SALAD WITH MAPLE		SUNFLOWER POPPY SEED	
SYRUP VINAIGRETTE	88	MUFFINS	69
NUTTY ORANGE PANCAKES	65	SUPER YUMMY GRILLED	
ORZO SALAD	51	SANDWICH	111
OVERNIGHT OATS		TOMATO-POTATO-ZUCCHINI	
WITH FRUIT	109	TIAN	101
PAN-FRIED SALMON FILLET		TROPICAL OATMEAL	112
FOR 2 WITH DILL SAUCE	79	TUNA-STUFFED PEPPERS	
PEAS & NOODLES		FOR TWO	80
PARMIGIANO	98	VEGETABLE FRITTATA	
PIÑA COLADA SLUSH	30	WITH GREENS	78
PORK TENDERLOIN		WILD PLUM TEA	33
WITH ROASTED		WILD RICE PANCAKES	113
APPLES & ONIONS	85	ZUCCHINI-APRICOT/	
POTATO HASH WITH OKRA	99	RAISIN SALAD	56
QUINOA & HONEY		ZUCCHINI & CARROT	
BEET SALAD	42	STRANDS	57
RASPBERRY SMOOTHIE	31		
RASPBERRY SMOOTHIE BOWL	66		
RASPBERRY-PEACH SALAD	52		
RICE & WALNUTS	110		
ROASTED APPLE SAUCE	53		
ROASTED PUMPKIN SEEDS	67		
ROASTED STONE-FRUIT FOR 2	68		
ROSY CRANBERRY PUNCH	32		

Acknowledgements

After God, who guides my life, I wish to thank my family, especially my husband for supporting all my endeavors. Special thanks need to be given to my sister, Jo Fry and my son, Robert Pizza for their technical and grammatical expertise. And, to my daughter, Andrea Pojman for her quiet, never-wavering support.

I want to thank all my medical caregivers, by name, for their expert care throughout the years:

Dr. Perin Alfred and his staff at Pulmonary Physicians PA in Ocala, FL.

Dr. William Cole, Brandon Brown, NP-C, Pamela Wright, APN and their staff at LeConte Pulmonary & Critical Care Medicine, Sevierville, TN.

Dr. Nidhi Kaul at Ocala Health Family Care Specialists, Ocala FL

Dr. Eric Littleton at UT Primary Care in Sevierville, TN

And, the professionals at:

LeConte Medical Center's Cardiac and Pulmonary Rehabilitation, Sevierville, TN and Munroe Regional Medical Center Cardiopulmonary Rehab, Ocala, FL

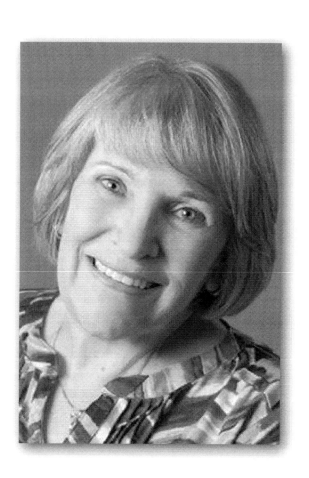

About the Author

Teri Pizza is a columnist, speaker and author of several books. She attributes living the *Eat to Breathe Plan* and her fabulous team of medical professionals for her ability to live a viable life while battling COPD. "Not quite as active as pre-COPD but very close!"

In addition to writing and speaking, she enjoys her crazy-crabby cat, Holly Berry, as well as cooking, reading and being with her husband, John. They divide their time between Gatlinburg, TN and Ocala, FL with frequent trips to visit family in Illinois and Wisconsin.

Let Teri know what you think of her book. Leave a review at Amazon.com or drop her an email at tnmntlady@gmail.com.

All of Teri Pizza's books are available from Amazon.com.

Made in the USA
Charleston, SC
06 March 2017